Vaccines Exposed: Empowering Communities to Overcome Vaccine Hesitancy

Table of Contents

Vaccines have been one of humanity's most powerful tools against disease, saving millions of lives and transforming public health. Yet for many minority communities, vaccines remain a source of uncertainty, mistrust, and unanswered questions. Historical injustices, systemic barriers, and cultural differences have created a divide between the promise of vaccines and the trust needed to embrace them fully.

This book, *Vaccines Exposed*, is a guide to understanding the truth about vaccines, addressing the fears and skepticism that persist, and empowering healthcare professionals and community leaders to foster trust in vaccination. It is written with a clear purpose: to expose not only the science and history behind vaccines but also the social challenges that prevent their full acceptance in communities that have too often been underserved.

Vaccines are not just medical interventions—they are shields against illness, tools of hope, and acts of communal responsibility. They protect not only the person vaccinated but also the most vulnerable among us, such as infants and those with compromised immune systems. Diseases like smallpox, which once ravaged humanity, have been eradicated through vaccines. Others, like polio and measles, are now rare thanks to widespread immunization. These successes remind us of what's possible when communities come together to embrace the lifesaving power of vaccines.

For minority communities, vaccine hesitancy often has roots that go deeper than scientific skepticism. Historical abuses, such as the Tuskegee Syphilis Study and the exploitation of Henrietta Lacks, have left scars that linger today. Systemic inequities, including healthcare deserts and language barriers, further hinder access and trust. The spread of misinformation on social media and by word of mouth only compounds these issues, creating fear and confusion.

Healthcare professionals and community leaders are uniquely positioned to bridge this gap. By addressing concerns with empathy, providing culturally relevant education, and building trust, they can create meaningful change. *Vaccines Exposed* equips you with the knowledge and tools to take on this critical challenge.

This book is not about persuasion through force or judgment. It is about equipping people with the facts they need to make informed decisions. It is about building connections and trust. And it is about ensuring that every child, every family, and every community has access to the protection that vaccines offer.

Thank you for joining me on this journey. Together, we can expose the truth about vaccines, address the doubts that hold people back, and create healthier, more equitable communities for all.

Chapter 1: What Are Vaccines?

Vaccines are one of the greatest medical achievements in history. They have saved countless lives, reduced the burden of infectious diseases, and transformed how humanity combats epidemics. But understanding what vaccines are and how they work is essential to appreciating their importance and addressing the fears that surround them.

A vaccine is a medical product that prepares your immune system to fight harmful germs, such as viruses or bacteria, before they can make you sick. Unlike medications that treat diseases after they occur, vaccines are preventative, arming your body with the tools it needs to stop infections before they happen.

Vaccines work by mimicking an infection. They contain harmless versions of germs—or parts of germs—that trigger the body's immune response. This process teaches your immune system how to recognize and fight the real germ if you are ever exposed to it.

When you receive a vaccine, your body creates antibodies—special proteins that attack the germ—and stores this knowledge in its immune memory. The next time you encounter the germ, your body can respond quickly and effectively, preventing you from getting sick.

Vaccines come in different types, each tailored to fight specific diseases. Some of the most common types include:

- **Live Attenuated Vaccines**: These contain weakened versions of the germ that cannot cause disease in healthy people. Examples include the measles, mumps, and rubella (MMR) vaccine and the chickenpox vaccine.
- **Inactivated Vaccines**: These use germs that have been killed, ensuring they cannot cause disease. The polio vaccine is an example.
- **Subunit Vaccines**: These include only specific parts of the germ, such as proteins. The human papillomavirus (HPV) vaccine and hepatitis B vaccine fall into this category.
- **mRNA Vaccines**: These teach your cells to produce a harmless piece of the germ, triggering an immune response. The Pfizer-BioNTech and Moderna COVID-19 vaccines use this groundbreaking technology.

Vaccines are carefully designed to be both safe and effective, providing immunity without causing the illness itself.

Vaccines are essential for preventing some of the world's most dangerous diseases. Before vaccines, diseases like smallpox, polio, and measles caused widespread suffering and death. Today, smallpox has been eradicated globally, polio is nearly eliminated, and measles cases have drastically declined in areas with high vaccination rates.

When enough people are vaccinated, communities achieve something called **herd immunity**. This means that even people who cannot be vaccinated—like newborns or those with certain medical conditions—are protected because the disease has fewer opportunities to spread. Herd immunity is crucial for preventing outbreaks and protecting the most vulnerable members of society.

Vaccines do more than protect individuals—they benefit entire communities and generations. Diseases that once struck fear into families, such as diphtheria and tetanus, are now rare thanks to vaccines. However, maintaining high vaccination rates is critical. In areas where vaccine coverage drops, diseases can make a comeback, as seen in recent measles outbreaks in parts of the world.

Understanding the science of vaccines is the first step in addressing concerns and building trust. Vaccines are not just about preventing illness; they are about ensuring a healthier, safer future for everyone.

In the next chapter, we will address the myths and misconceptions that often fuel vaccine hesitancy, separating fact from fiction.

Chapter 2: Vaccine Myths vs. Facts

Misinformation about vaccines is widespread and can create fear and doubt. This chapter addresses some of the most common myths surrounding vaccines, providing clear and evidence-based facts to help separate truth from fiction.

Myth 1: Vaccines Cause Autism

This myth stems from a 1998 study by Dr. Andrew Wakefield, which falsely claimed a link between the MMR (measles, mumps, and rubella) vaccine and autism. The study was later discredited and retracted by the journal that published it. Wakefield lost his medical license for misconduct.

Since then, numerous large-scale studies have found no connection between vaccines and autism. For example, a 2019 Danish study involving over 650,000 children conclusively showed that the MMR vaccine does not increase the risk of autism. Vaccines remain one of the safest medical interventions available.

Myth 2: Natural Immunity is Better than Vaccination

Some people believe that contracting a disease and recovering provides stronger immunity than a vaccine. While natural immunity can be robust, it comes at a high cost. Diseases like measles, polio, and COVID-19 can lead to severe complications, long-term health issues, or even death.

Vaccines provide immunity without the risks of severe illness. For example, the HPV vaccine prevents infections that can lead to cervical cancer, and the measles vaccine protects against brain swelling (encephalitis), which can result from natural infection. Choosing vaccination means choosing protection without unnecessary suffering.

Myth 3: Vaccines Contain Dangerous Ingredients

Concerns about vaccine ingredients are common, but it's important to understand that all components in vaccines serve a purpose and are used in safe amounts.

- **Aluminum**: Used to boost the immune response. The amount in vaccines is much lower than what we encounter daily through food and water.
- **Thimerosal**: A mercury-based preservative that has been removed from most vaccines since 2001, except in multi-dose flu vials. Studies show it is safe in the small amounts used.
- **Formaldehyde**: Used to inactivate viruses and toxins during production. Our bodies naturally produce far more formaldehyde than is present in any vaccine.

Each ingredient undergoes rigorous testing to ensure safety.

Myth 4: Vaccines Aren't Necessary Anymore

Many vaccine-preventable diseases have become rare in some parts of the world, leading people to believe vaccines are no longer necessary.

However, these diseases are rare because of high vaccination rates. If those rates decline, the diseases can return.

For example, measles outbreaks have occurred in communities with low vaccination rates, even in countries where the disease was previously under control. In 2019, over 200,000 deaths worldwide were attributed to measles—a disease that is preventable with vaccination. Vaccines remain essential to keep these diseases at bay.

Myth 5: Vaccines Overload the Immune System

Some people worry that receiving multiple vaccines at once overwhelms the immune system. In reality, the immune system encounters thousands of antigens (substances that trigger an immune response) every day. Vaccines introduce only a tiny fraction of that number.

Vaccines are designed to work together, and studies show that receiving multiple vaccines during a single visit is safe and effective. Combining vaccines, such as the DTaP vaccine (diphtheria, tetanus, and pertussis), reduces the number of shots needed while providing strong protection.

Myth 6: Vaccines Were Rushed and Are Unsafe

COVID-19 vaccines, in particular, have faced criticism for being developed "too quickly." While it's true that these vaccines were developed in record time, they still underwent rigorous testing. The speed was due to decades of prior research on mRNA technology, global collaboration, and unprecedented funding.

Tens of thousands of participants were involved in clinical trials, and safety continues to be monitored through systems like VAERS (Vaccine Adverse Event Reporting System). The rapid development did not compromise safety or effectiveness.

Myth 7: Vaccines Cause Severe Side Effects

Most vaccine side effects are mild, such as a sore arm or low fever, and they usually go away within a day or two. Severe reactions, like anaphylaxis, are extremely rare—occurring in about 1 in a million doses—and are treatable.

The benefits of vaccines far outweigh the risks. For example, the risk of complications from measles is far higher than any risk posed by the MMR vaccine.

Misinformation can spread quickly, especially on social media, where false claims often go viral. Addressing myths with evidence and empathy is crucial to building trust in vaccines. By sharing the facts, we can empower individuals to make informed decisions and protect their communities.

In the next chapter, we'll explore the unique challenges and historical factors that contribute to vaccine hesitancy in minority communities and discuss strategies to address these issues effectively.

Chapter 3: Vaccines and Minority Communities

Vaccines have the power to protect lives and prevent suffering, but in many minority communities, they are met with skepticism. This hesitancy is often rooted in historical injustices, systemic inequities, and cultural barriers. Addressing these challenges requires understanding the unique concerns of these communities and working collaboratively to rebuild trust.

For many minority groups, mistrust of vaccines is tied to a long history of unethical medical practices. The Tuskegee Syphilis Study, conducted from 1932 to 1972, is a painful example. In this study, Black men with syphilis were deliberately left untreated so researchers could observe the progression of the disease, even after penicillin became available. Similarly, the story of Henrietta Lacks, whose cells were taken without her consent and used for groundbreaking research, highlights how minority communities have often been exploited by the medical system.

These historical injustices have left scars that persist across generations, fostering distrust in healthcare institutions. This mistrust is not just historical; systemic inequities continue to limit access to quality healthcare in many minority communities. Healthcare deserts, where clinics and hospitals are scarce, make vaccination harder to access. Language barriers, cultural differences, and financial challenges further complicate efforts to vaccinate underserved populations.

Misinformation adds another layer of complexity. False claims about vaccines often spread faster in communities that already feel marginalized. Social media and targeted disinformation campaigns exploit existing fears, making it even harder to combat myths and encourage vaccination.

Despite these challenges, there are success stories that show how trust can be rebuilt. During the COVID-19 pandemic, partnerships with Black churches proved effective in increasing vaccination rates in African American communities. These initiatives worked because they were led by trusted community leaders who addressed concerns with empathy and understanding.

Similarly, Hispanic outreach programs have shown success by providing bilingual materials and partnering with schools to educate parents about the HPV vaccine. Native American communities achieved high COVID-19 vaccination rates by integrating traditional practices and involving tribal leaders in the decision-making process. These examples highlight the importance of culturally tailored approaches that respect the values and needs of each community.

Improving vaccine uptake in minority communities requires more than just education; it demands action to address systemic barriers. Mobile clinics, free vaccinations, and culturally relevant outreach programs are essential steps. Empowering community leaders, pastors, and local advocates to champion vaccination efforts can make a significant impact.

As healthcare professionals and community leaders work to build trust, it's important to acknowledge past injustices openly and demonstrate a commitment to ethical practices. Transparency, empathy, and collaboration are the keys to bridging the gap between skepticism and acceptance.

By understanding the unique challenges faced by minority communities, we can create targeted strategies to improve vaccination rates and protect the health of all individuals, regardless of their background.

In the next chapter, we will explore the rigorous process by which vaccines are developed and tested, demonstrating why they are among the safest medical interventions available.

Chapter 4: How Vaccines Are Made and Tested

Vaccines are among the safest and most rigorously tested medical interventions. Before they are approved for use, vaccines undergo years of research, testing, and monitoring to ensure their safety and effectiveness. Understanding this process is crucial to building confidence in vaccines, especially in communities where skepticism persists.

The journey of a vaccine begins with research. Scientists study the disease-causing germ—whether a virus, bacteria, or toxin—and identify the part of it that triggers the immune system. This could be a specific protein, a sugar, or even the whole germ, in a weakened or inactivated form. Early research often involves laboratory studies and animal testing to assess potential effectiveness and safety.

If a vaccine candidate shows promise in the lab, it moves on to preclinical testing, where researchers gather data to determine whether it is safe enough to be tested in humans. Only a small fraction of vaccine candidates make it past this stage.

The next step is clinical trials, which take place in three carefully monitored phases:

- **Phase 1**: A small group of healthy volunteers (20–100 people) receives the vaccine. The focus is on safety, identifying any immediate side effects, and determining the correct dose.
- **Phase 2**: Hundreds of participants are involved, including people from the target population (e.g., children, older adults). This phase assesses safety further and evaluates how well the vaccine stimulates an immune response.
- **Phase 3**: Thousands to tens of thousands of participants are recruited to confirm the vaccine's safety and effectiveness. This phase often uses randomized controlled trials, where some participants receive the vaccine and others receive a placebo. Researchers compare the outcomes to determine how well the vaccine works in preventing disease.

Once clinical trials are complete, the vaccine manufacturer submits all data to regulatory agencies, such as the FDA in the United States or the EMA in Europe. These agencies rigorously review the evidence before approving or licensing the vaccine. Only vaccines that meet strict safety and efficacy standards are approved for use.

Even after approval, vaccines are closely monitored through post-marketing surveillance systems like VAERS (Vaccine Adverse Event Reporting System) in the U.S. This ongoing monitoring ensures that any rare or long-term side effects are quickly identified and addressed.

The speed at which COVID-19 vaccines were developed has raised concerns, but it's important to understand that the rapid timeline was made possible by years of prior research on mRNA technology, massive global collaboration, and overlapping trial phases. Safety was never compromised, as the vaccines underwent the same rigorous testing as any other vaccine.

Transparency and accountability are central to the vaccine development process. Independent advisory committees, like the Advisory Committee on Immunization Practices (ACIP), review the data and make recommendations to ensure public confidence.

Vaccines are held to higher safety standards than most other medical products because they are given to healthy individuals to prevent disease, not to treat illness. This is why every step of the development process is designed to minimize risk and maximize benefits.

Understanding how vaccines are made and tested is essential for addressing fears and skepticism. When people see the rigorous scientific process behind vaccines, they can trust that these life-saving tools are safe and effective.

In the next chapter, we'll explore strategies for overcoming vaccine hesitancy, with a focus on empathetic communication and community engagement.

Chapter 5: Overcoming Vaccine Hesitancy

Vaccine hesitancy is a significant barrier to achieving widespread immunization, especially in communities that have experienced historical injustices or systemic neglect. Addressing these concerns requires empathy, cultural sensitivity, and evidence-based strategies to foster trust and understanding.

Vaccine hesitancy is often rooted in fear, misinformation, or personal experiences that shape people's perceptions of healthcare. Some may worry about vaccine safety, while others distrust the institutions that recommend vaccination. In minority communities, hesitancy is frequently tied to historical exploitation, such as the Tuskegee Syphilis Study, and ongoing disparities in access to quality healthcare.

Misinformation plays a major role in reinforcing doubts. False claims, often amplified by social media, create confusion and fear. For example, myths linking vaccines to infertility or severe side effects persist despite being repeatedly debunked. Addressing these misconceptions requires clear and accessible communication tailored to the audience's needs.

Empathy is the foundation of effective communication about vaccines. People who are hesitant are not necessarily "anti-vaccine"—many are simply unsure and have unanswered questions. Listening without judgment and validating their concerns is the first step in building trust. Healthcare professionals and community leaders must approach these conversations with respect and an open mind, offering factual information while addressing fears with compassion.

Community engagement is another essential strategy. Minority communities often place greater trust in local leaders, such as pastors, teachers, and grassroots organizers, than in unfamiliar healthcare providers or government agencies. Partnering with these trusted figures can help amplify accurate vaccine information and encourage participation. For example, vaccination clinics held in churches during the COVID-19 pandemic successfully increased uptake in African American communities by combining familiar spaces with trusted voices.

Cultural relevance is key to effective outreach. Educational materials should reflect the values, language, and priorities of the community they serve. In Hispanic communities, for instance, bilingual resources and family-focused messaging have been successful in promoting vaccines like HPV. Similarly, Native American tribes have incorporated traditional practices and tribal leaders into vaccination campaigns, achieving some of the highest COVID-19 vaccination rates in the U.S.

Improving accessibility is equally important. Logistical barriers, such as transportation issues, long wait times, or lack of nearby clinics, can discourage people from getting vaccinated. Solutions like mobile clinics, extended hours, and vaccination events in community centers can remove these obstacles and make vaccines more convenient to access.

Combatting misinformation requires proactive efforts to share accurate and engaging information. Social media campaigns, community workshops, and Q&A sessions with trusted healthcare providers can help counter myths and build confidence. Encouraging critical thinking and teaching people how to identify reliable sources of information is another powerful way to fight misinformation.

Healthcare professionals have a unique responsibility to address vaccine hesitancy with patience and understanding. Using techniques like motivational interviewing—asking open-ended questions, exploring concerns, and collaboratively setting goals—can help guide hesitant patients toward informed decisions.

Ultimately, overcoming vaccine hesitancy is about more than correcting myths; it's about building relationships and addressing systemic inequities. By investing in education, accessibility, and trust-building, we can ensure that everyone—regardless of their background—has the opportunity to benefit from life-saving vaccines.

In the next chapter, we'll look to the future of vaccines, exploring groundbreaking advances in technology and the potential for vaccines to address not just infectious diseases, but also cancer, Alzheimer's, and more.

Chapter 6: The Future of Vaccines

Vaccines have already changed the world, eradicating smallpox, nearly eliminating polio, and protecting billions from deadly diseases. But the future holds even greater promise. Advances in science and technology are paving the way for vaccines that could prevent new illnesses, improve global health equity, and address conditions far beyond infectious diseases.

One of the most exciting developments in vaccine technology is the use of messenger RNA (mRNA) platforms. These vaccines, such as the Pfizer-BioNTech and Moderna COVID-19 vaccines, work by instructing cells to produce a harmless piece of the virus, triggering an immune response. Unlike traditional vaccines, mRNA vaccines can be developed quickly and adjusted easily to address new variants or emerging diseases. Researchers are now exploring mRNA vaccines for HIV, influenza, and even cancer.

DNA vaccines are another promising innovation. Similar to mRNA vaccines, they provide genetic instructions for the immune system to recognize and fight pathogens. DNA vaccines are stable at higher temperatures, making them easier to store and distribute in low-resource settings. Current trials are investigating their potential to combat diseases like Zika virus, hepatitis, and some cancers.

Nanoparticle vaccines are also on the horizon. These tiny particles mimic the structure of viruses, making them highly effective at stimulating the immune system. They can be tailored to target specific diseases, such as malaria and tuberculosis, which remain major global health challenges.

Beyond infectious diseases, vaccines are expanding into entirely new areas. Cancer vaccines, for example, aim to prevent or treat certain types of cancer by targeting the abnormal cells that cause the disease. The HPV vaccine already prevents cervical and other cancers linked to the human papillomavirus, and researchers are developing therapeutic vaccines for melanoma, breast cancer, and lung cancer.

Vaccines for neurodegenerative diseases, like Alzheimer's, are another area of groundbreaking research. These vaccines target harmful proteins in the brain that contribute to memory loss and cognitive decline. Though still in experimental stages, they hold the potential to revolutionize how we approach aging-related diseases.

Innovations in vaccine delivery are also shaping the future. Microneedle patches, which deliver vaccines through the skin without the need for needles, promise a painless and convenient option that eliminates the fear of injections. Oral and inhalable vaccines are being developed for diseases like COVID-19 and tuberculosis, offering easier administration and increased accessibility.

Global health equity is at the heart of many of these advancements. Thermostable vaccines that don't require refrigeration could transform vaccination efforts in remote areas, reducing reliance on cold storage systems. Self-amplifying RNA (saRNA) technology, which allows for lower doses and faster production, could make vaccines more affordable and accessible worldwide.

Preparing for the next pandemic is another key focus for the future of vaccines. Researchers are developing pan-virus vaccines, which target entire families of viruses rather than individual strains. This approach could provide long-lasting protection against multiple pathogens, reducing the risk of future outbreaks. Predictive analytics and artificial intelligence are also being used to identify potential pandemics early, allowing vaccine development to begin before a crisis occurs.

Despite these exciting advancements, challenges remain. Ethical considerations, such as ensuring equitable distribution and addressing vaccine hesitancy, will be critical. The rapid pace of innovation must also be balanced with thorough safety testing to maintain public trust.

The future of vaccines is bright, but its success depends on global collaboration and shared commitment. From eradicating diseases in low-income countries to developing vaccines for cancer and Alzheimer's, the possibilities are endless. With continued investment in research, innovation, and equity, vaccines will remain one of the most powerful tools for improving health and saving lives.

In the final chapter, we'll summarize the key lessons of this book and discuss how you can take action to promote vaccines in your community and beyond.

A Call to Action

Vaccines are one of the greatest achievements of modern medicine, saving lives and protecting communities from deadly diseases. Yet, their success relies on trust, understanding, and collective action. This book has explored the science of vaccines, debunked myths, addressed the roots of vaccine hesitancy, and highlighted the unique challenges faced by minority communities. Now, it's time to take what we've learned and turn it into action.

Vaccines are more than individual choices—they are a shared responsibility. Every vaccination helps protect those who cannot be vaccinated, such as newborns, cancer patients, and individuals with weakened immune systems. By getting vaccinated, we contribute to herd immunity, reducing the spread of disease and saving lives. This is especially crucial in minority communities, where systemic barriers and historical mistrust have left gaps in vaccine coverage.

Healthcare professionals, community leaders, and advocates have a vital role to play in overcoming these challenges. By listening with empathy, addressing fears with evidence, and creating culturally relevant solutions, we can build trust and increase vaccine confidence. We must also acknowledge and address systemic inequities, ensuring that every community has access to the vaccines and healthcare services they need.

Education is one of the most powerful tools we have. Sharing reliable, evidence-based information about vaccines can combat misinformation and empower individuals to make informed decisions. This means engaging with hesitant individuals without judgment, providing clear and accessible resources, and partnering with trusted voices in the community.

Action is equally important. Advocate for policies that improve vaccine accessibility, such as mobile clinics, extended hours, and affordable immunization programs. Support organizations that work to bring vaccines to underserved areas, both locally and globally. Encourage conversations about vaccines in schools, places of worship, and community centers, making vaccination a shared goal.

The future of vaccines holds incredible promise, with new technologies and innovations that will save even more lives. But that future depends on us—on our ability to build trust, spread awareness, and ensure that vaccines reach every corner of the world.

This is not just a book about vaccines; it's a call to action. Each of us has the power to make a difference, whether by vaccinating ourselves and our families, sharing knowledge with others, or advocating for equity in healthcare. Together, we can protect lives, build trust, and create a healthier, safer future for all.

Thank you for joining me on this journey. Let's take the next step—together.

References

Below is a list of references that provide the scientific evidence, historical context, and expert recommendations mentioned throughout the book. These trusted sources will help readers explore the topics further and build confidence in the credibility of the information presented.

Peer-Reviewed Studies and Reviews

1. Graña C., Ghosn L., Evrenoglou T., et al. (2022). *Efficacy and safety of COVID-19 vaccines: A systematic review.* Cochrane Database of Systematic Reviews. Retrieved from Cochrane Library.
2. Madsen, K.M., Hviid, A., Vestergaard, M., et al. (2002). *A population-based study of measles, mumps, and rubella vaccination and autism.* The New England Journal of Medicine, 347(19), 1477-1482.
3. Wakefield, A.J., Murch, S.H., Anthony, A., et al. (1998). *Ileal-lymphoid-nodular hyperplasia, non-specific colitis, and pervasive developmental disorder in children.* The Lancet. (Retracted).
4. Jefferson, T., Del Mar, C., Foxlee, R., et al. (2023). *Physical interventions to interrupt or reduce the spread of respiratory viruses.* Cochrane Database of Systematic Reviews. Retrieved from Cochrane Library.
5. Plotkin, S.A., Orenstein, W.A., Offit, P.A., & Edwards, K.M. (2018). *Plotkin's Vaccines* (7th ed.). Elsevier.

Official Organizations and Reports

6. Centers for Disease Control and Prevention (CDC). (2023). *Vaccines and immunizations.* Retrieved from https://www.cdc.gov/vaccines.

7. World Health Organization (WHO). (2023). *Global vaccine safety and efficacy.* Retrieved from https://www.who.int.

8. Vaccine Adverse Event Reporting System (VAERS). (2023). *Data and monitoring systems.* Retrieved from https://vaers.hhs.gov.

9. Gavi, the Vaccine Alliance. (2023). *Equitable access to vaccines.* Retrieved from https://www.gavi.org.

10. Advisory Committee on Immunization Practices (ACIP). (2023). *Recommendations on vaccine safety.* Retrieved from https://www.cdc.gov/vaccines/acip.

Books and Articles

11. Offit, P.A. (2013). *Deadly Choices: How the Anti-Vaccine Movement Threatens Us All.* Basic Books.

12. Paul, O.F. (2015). *Vaccinated: One Man's Quest to Defeat the World's Deadliest Diseases.* Harper.

13. Glanz, J.M., Wagner, N.M., Narwaney, K.J., et al. (2013). *A mixed methods study of parental vaccine hesitancy.* Journal of Pediatrics, 164(3), 610-616.

Web-Based Educational Resources

14. Cochrane Library. (2023). *Evidence-based reviews on vaccine safety and efficacy.* Retrieved from https://www.cochranelibrary.com.

15. ClinicalTrials.gov. (2023). *Ongoing vaccine trials and results.* Retrieved from https://clinicaltrials.gov.

16. Immunization Action Coalition. (2023). *Vaccine information for healthcare professionals and the public.* Retrieved from https://www.immunize.org.